LIFE HISTORY ALBUM

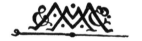

LIFE HISTORY ALBUM

TABLES AND CHARTS FOR RE-
CORDING THE DEVELOPMENT
OF BODY AND MIND FROM
CHILDHOOD UPWARDS, WITH
INTRODUCTORY REMARKS

SECOND EDITION

REARRANGED BY

FRANCIS GALTON, D.C.L., F.R.S.

CAMBRIDGE UNIVERSITY PRESS

C. F. CLAY, Manager

LONDON: FETTER LANE, E.C.   EDINBURGH: 100, PRINCES STREET

H. K. LEWIS, 136, GOWER STREET, LONDON, W.C.
WILLIAM WESLEY AND SON, 28, ESSEX STREET,
LONDON, W.C.
CHICAGO: UNIVERSITY OF CHICAGO PRESS

BOMBAY, CALCUTTA AND MADRAS:
MACMILLAN AND CO., LIMITED
TORONTO: J. M. DENT AND SONS, LIMITED
TOKYO: THE MARUZEN-KABUSHIKI-KAISHA

1902

CAMBRIDGE UNIVERSITY PRESS
Cambridge, New York, Melbourne, Madrid, Cape Town,
Singapore, São Paulo, Delhi, Mexico City

Cambridge University Press
The Edinburgh Building, Cambridge CB2 8RU, UK

Published in the United States of America by Cambridge University Press, New York

www.cambridge.org
Information on this title: www.cambridge.org/9781107632141

First published 1902
First paperback edition 2013

A catalogue record for this publication is available from the British Library

ISBN 978-1-107-63214-1 Paperback

LIFE HISTORY ALBUM

Containing the Records of the Life of

NAME ....

BORN ....

AT ....

CONTENTS

B

PREFACE

THE first appearance of the *Life History Album* many years ago was due to the enthusiasm of the late Dr. Mahomed, then a medical man of much promise, and· apparently on the point of rising to considerable eminence in his profession. He had firmly persuaded himself that some such work would be favoured and promoted by medical men throughout the country if it were composed under the eyes of physicians growing into repute in the medical world, and if it were afterwards strongly recommended, as it probably would be, by the Collective Investigation Committee of the Medical Association, of which he was an active member. He made it a further condition that my name should appear as its editor, I being known at that time to be much occupied in such matters. To this I agreed with some reluctance, for I wished to bear the entire responsibility or none at all. So a small committee of medical men was formed who met frequently at my house, where the book was mostly composed. But the result did not at all satisfy myself, neither do I think that it satisfied the others. It was too bulky and ill arranged. In fact it was emphatically a case of too many cooks. Each had his own views, and I believe that any one of us acting alone would have produced a better balanced book than we did working together. Soon after it was in print Dr. Mahomed contracted typhoid fever, the very subject of his own special studies, and he died, to the great regret of myself and of many others. The tributes of affection to his memory from his colleagues at Guy's Hospital were remarkable for their warmth and high appreciation of his ability. He being gone, none of the remaining medical members of the committee concerned themselves much further with the work, and the main part of Dr. Mahomed's scheme was never fulfilled. However, the book had a small circulation, until of late years it fell out of print. Being frequently urged by friends whose opinion I trust, to largely re-arrange and re-write it, I have at length done so—with what success those who may use it will judge.

F. G.

INTRODUCTORY REMARKS

THIS Album is intended for the use of persons of any age, however advanced, who may be inclined to begin to use it. They would have to supply records of past years as they best could, partly from their own memories and notes, partly from those of others, and thenceforward to keep the register up to date. Though their books would be incompletely filled, they would be of considerable interest, and certainly very much better than no record at all. Any one of them might serve as groundwork for an autobiography.

This book is, however, especially suitable as a present in readiness for infants expected to be born, or for very young children, with the understanding that it should remain in charge of the parents for many years, who would make the necessary entries during that time. As soon as the child had grown old enough to appreciate its importance and to take charge of it, it would be handed over to him or her.

In fulfilment of this two-fold purpose the Album contains tables suitable for every year from birth to extreme old age. It is possible in some few cases that the same book may be used as a register during the whole of a lifetime, because a fraction of the population—small relatively, but considerable in absolute numbers—are naturally disposed to register events methodically. Some of these may continue to make records to the end of their lives in the very same Album that their parents had initiated for them.

The wider the span of the record, the more instructive it will be; but the scrappiest of registers will prove of interest, and it may be of considerable utility to its owner.

The merit claimed for this Album is that it presents whatever it contains in an orderly fashion, and that while it affords space enough for essentials, it discourages prolixity. The amount of important information that one of these Albums could hold is very large. The five or six lines allotted to each year are enough for an adequate notice of its leading events; but if the year should have been an exceptionally eventful one, room is provided in blank spaces for additional remarks.

The Medical History and the Anthropometric Observations taken together, will supply a complete biological history up to date, which might frequently become an invaluable guide in determining future conduct. By turning over the pages of the book the main landmarks of the owner's past life will successively come under review in their true sequence and in their just proportions. His chief hereditary predispositions can be seen at a single opening of its pages 1 2, 1 3. The trials that his constitution may have undergone, through illness or over-fatigue of mind or body, are duly recorded, and their after effects as well. The good or bad influences of change in habit, diet, residence, and so forth, may be traced out. The progress of development, with its occasional arrests, is clearly pictured in the Charts of weight and stature. While the entries are proceeding, the insidious approach of preventable maladies may be detected and thwarted. An excellent example of this may be expected often to occur in the case of incipient short-sightedness, induced when at school by poring over books or writing in an ill-disposed light and in faulty attitudes. Finally, a well-filled Album is eminently worthy of becoming an heir-loom, being filled with comforts and warnings to generations yet to come.

The future of each man is mainly a direct consequence of the past— of his own biological history, and of those of his ancestors. It is therefore of high importance when planning for the future to keep the past under frequent review, all in its just proportion, and this is exactly what this Album is intended to help him to do.

Memory alone is an imperfect and deceitful guide ; it preserves only a trifling part of the events of early life, and that part far from correctly. The extreme vividness with which a few childish incidents are usually recalled gives a very exaggerated view of the power of its grasp. Anybody who attempts to compile a sustained history of his early years will soon be persuaded of the truth of this remark, for he will surely become aware of huge gaps of time that he is totally unable to give account of. Every autobiography that I have seen testifies to these lapses of memory. Again, when one happens to meet a friend not seen since early life, and to compare recollections, it is astonishing to find how differently the two memories have behaved. The one man fails to recall a multitude of events that have strongly impressed the other. Even as to those they alike remember as wholes, it will often occur that their memories disagree in essential details. In fact, the experience gained by such interviews is commonly humiliating to both.

It is too much to expect that even the most scrupulously kept records will be written throughout with perfect veracity. Healthily minded persons are seldom disposed to lay themselves wholly bare in written words. There will be omissions in every Album, sometimes of matters of fact and at other times of the real inwardness of events, that are of high importance to the right understanding of a life history. The writer of the Album will mentally supply the omissions and interpret the misleading euphemisms when he refers to its pages ; other persons who read his records must be prepared for their existence. Thus in matters of disease, an unsurmountable prejudice exists in many sensitive persons against ascribing cancer and insanity to their ancestors in direct terms. They shrink from the thought of recording hereditary possibilities that might destroy the peace of mind of their descendants, and perhaps work their own fulfilment. The duty of parents to be truthful historiographers seems overborne by what they consider to be a still more pressing duty to their children. It is almost useless to attempt to calm hypersensitive feelings by pointing to the fact that healthful tendencies are just as heritable as morbid ones, and that every child is sure to be endowed with both. So I will confine myself to the mention of an instructive experience of my own, which was gained while working at the family histories of a multitude of individuals. They were so tabulated that the medical history of any individual could be concealed by the hand, or by a sheet of paper, while those of all his immediate ancestors, namely, parents, grand-parents, uncles, and aunts, were exposed. I experimented frequently in guessing at the cause of death of a deceased individual from the knowledge of those of his ancestry, and I found my guesses to be on the whole grossly incorrect. But though the stated cause of death could not be predicted with any approach to a useful degree of accuracy, the inheritance of minor ailments was conspicuously manifest. For this reason, some stress is laid in the Album upon recording them. For my own part, I find no valid reason why the diseases of ancestors should be described otherwise than with perfect honesty, especially as a knowledge of them may induce their descendants to take reasonable precautions against inborn tendencies, instead of taking no precautions at all and doing themselves irreparable injury out of pure ignorance.

I will now explain in detail the ways in which it is intended that the Album should be filled.

Name and Initials.—It is intended that the name of the owner should be written in ink on the outside of the cover after the word "of," and that his or her initials should be similarly written on its back.

Method of Writing.—Write, in the first instance, very lightly with a soft and finely pointed pencil, and in small clear characters. Revise carefully, rubbing out where needed. When quite satisfied, go over the pencillings in ink, using a finely pointed pen. Lastly, rub out the pencil marks. Abundant room will be found for the entries if these directions are attended to. On the other hand, a page of handwriting that is crowded here, sprawls there, and is in part illegible, will be a reproach to the writer in after years whenever the book is opened at that place.

Genealogical Record.—The facts asked for under this heading only concern the Parents and Brothers and Sisters of the *Parents of the Owner* of the Album. If the owner be a child, this information will for the most part be easily obtained. Even then it is well to verify recollections and impressions by making inquiries from elderly relatives and family friends. But when the book is first taken in hand by a grown-up person on his own account, there will be more trouble in getting at the facts. The certified causes of death (not always to be depended on) are obtainable, by personal inquiry and a trifling fee, at the proper Government departments—namely, that of the Registrar-General, Somerset House, London, for deaths in England, and at the General Register Offices in Dublin and Edinburgh for those in Ireland and Scotland respectively. The deaths are registered according to the year of death, place, and name ; so, if the year of death be not exactly known, more than one volume must be consulted. Similarly if the place of death be doubtful.

The causes of death are apt to be incorrectly recorded in deference to the feelings of the parents, as mentioned above, secondary symptoms being registered instead of the primary ones. The more serious affections include gout, rheumatism, consumption, spitting of blood, struma (scrofula), cancer (and other forms of tumour), bronchitis, asthma, paralysis, epilepsy, insanity, heart-disease, dropsy of abdomen, general dropsy (Bright's disease), diabetes, stone, goitre, and fistula. The minor ailments which are well worth noting include colds in the head or throat, sick headaches, sleeplessness, boils, quinsy, enlarged glands in the neck, nose bleeding, bilious attacks (with particulars), constipation, skin eruptions, varicose veins, imperfections of sight, hearing, or dentition.

When the genealogy has been completed for any one member of a family of brothers and sisters, it can easily be copied into the books of other members, to every one of whom it is of like importance.

Family Characteristics.—The page that follows the Genealogy is intended to contain a notice of such marked characteristics as may be common to at least two (preferably to many more) members of the Father's and Mother's families respectively. Only those are asked for which would engage an intelligent stranger's attention as being distinctly interesting from a hereditary point of view. Characteristics of this kind are exceedingly various, and though clearly marked they may be trifling in themselves. They relate to stature, form, features, gestures, or voice ; to the growth of hair and its colour ; to eye colour ; and to aptitudes of all sorts, whether moral, æsthetic, or intellectual.

Description of Child at Birth.—The observations asked for are simple and easily made at the time. They are of interest in relation to future development. The eyes at birth are always dark blue, but usually begin to change their hue after a few days. Note when they do so, and to what colour.

As regards " Mother's Marks," the question has been allowed to stand in deference to a widely felt prejudice ; but, considering that the negative evidence of the existence of marks being due to mental impressions made on the mother before the birth of the child, is almost overwhelming, no credence can be expected to the statement of facts to the contrary unless they be substantiated by an exact transcript of notes made *before* the birth of the child.

Life and Medical History.—Stress has already been laid on small, clear handwriting, which is particularly appropriate here. It is not intended that these pages should contain more than brief summaries of the past year, made, say, on the birthday. Current notes, prescriptions, and the like may be stuffed into the pocket of the book until the time arrives for compiling the brief yearly retrospect. There is a little spare place left for Remarks, if any. The back of the entire page upon which the photographs are to be pasted might also be used for additional notes, and thin paper might be interleaved. More will be said a little further on, under a similar heading to the above, in reference to adult life. This may be read in advance.

Photographs, from Birth to Five Years of Age.—These will probably be of more interest as mementos of early childhood than of solid use. Still, on both accounts, some few of them should be preserved.

Weight and *Stature* will shortly be spoken of under the head of *Charts*.

After the close of the fifth year of age, more minute observations become feasible and important. The bulk of the Album therefore refers to these. The person's life is supposed to be divided into five-yearly terms, the first of which has already been dealt with. The remainder, up to extreme old age, are all scheduled in the same way. Eight pages are assigned to each five years. The first and second pages contain the Life and Medical History of each year. The third is left blank for Remarks, if any. The fourth and fifth are tabulated to hold Anthropometric Observations (which will be spoken of almost immediately), the sixth is blank, the seventh is for photographs, and the eighth is blank. Besides these, there are blank Charts waiting to be filled, which will be described shortly.

Life History.—What has been said under this heading concerning the period of childhood, applies equally to the rest of life ; but there is more to be added. A concise record is desirable of the main features of the person's history, habits, and surroundings during each year, so far as they may be exceptional, and of obvious interest or importance. No others are wanted. Each birthday would be a suitable opportunity for reviewing the events of the past year. Before beginning to write its summary, the following points should be successively considered, whether there be anything deserving of notice in respect to any one or more of them :—

1. *Place of residence.*—Change of residence, whether temporary or permanent.
2. *Occupation.*—Where carried on ; number of hours given to it.
3. *Recreations.*—Their character ; the number of hours given to them.
4. *Sleep.*—Its amount ; whether liable to be much disturbed.
5. *Food.*—Number of meals ; daily average of meat and alcohol.
6. *Anxiety.*—Whether much or none during the year ; its subject.
7. Any unusual *fatigue*, mental or bodily.
8. *Important Events*—as going to school or college, passing examinations, prizes, commencement of professional study, entering professional life or business, marriage, loss of near relations.

It must again be insisted that this formidable list is intended only as a reminder—not that remarks are wanted under each of its eight headings.

Medical History.—It is desirable, though it is not necessary, that these entries should be made or revised by a medical man. The points to be noticed are the duration of illness ; the number of days in which the person was incapacitated ; the nature of the maladies, and any peculiarity in their course ; their resultant effects, if marked ; and idiosyncrasies in respect to drugs and diet.

Anthropometric Observations.—As these cannot be made with advantage much before the time when the child is six years old, that is, at the end of his sixth year, the schedules in which they are to be entered are arranged to begin at that date. They are thenceforward continued for every year of life, so that a well-filled Album would show the development, the maximum limit, and afterwards the slow decay of the various faculties of the person to whom it refers. The term during which records are especially interesting is that of development, from childhood up to twenty-five years of age, when the broad tableland of maturity is reached. The sight and hearing should be tested frequently during youth, for it not uncommonly happens that children are blamed for carelessness and inattention when they are really suffering from defects in sight or hearing. Even so remarkable a deficiency as that of the sense of colour occasionally remains undetected until mature life. Dalton, the great chemist, who first drew attention to its existence, and from whom it receives its name, Daltonism, was an instance of this. It is said that he first became aware that his sight must be different to that of other men when, being a Quaker, he had selected a scarlet cloth as suitable material for his new drab coat, to the wonderment of his tailor. I have myself witnessed more than one painful discovery of the absence of colour sense in fully-grown youths who were tested at my laboratory. The importance of detecting incipient short-sightedness at school has already been dwelt upon.

The variety of anthropometric observations that might be of service is great, but easily accessible means do not yet exist for making them with precision, otherwise more would have been included in the schedule especially in respect to strength. Weight and stature are dealt with not here, but in the Charts about to be described; there is also room in these for entries as to strength and chest-girth when desired.

I hope that long before the lifetime of the incoming generation has closed, decimal measures will have superseded our present cumbrous and solitary system. If any of these Albums be then in existence, alterations may be made by hand in their headings.

Finger-prints.—Clear finger-prints, for possible service in future identification, can easily be secured by the end of the sixth year. Younger children are troublesome to deal with; but useful impressions may be got with patience even from babies. The prints should be made in printer's ink on thin paper, and a good example of them might be pasted on the first page under the owner's name. I do not know where the art of taking prints is regularly practised except in prisons. The way of doing it is explained in my book *Finger Prints* (Macmillan).

Photographs.—The seventh of the eight pages assigned to each five-yearly interval is for the reception of photographs made during that time. The sixth and eighth pages are blank, and might be utilised for the same purpose. The book is loosely bound to allow of this being occasionally done, so that photographs of residences, interiors, and other objects of biographical interest may be occasionally inserted.

The ideal portraiture for anthropological purposes is an exact full face and an exact profile, each one-seventh the size of nature. But the result is far from picturesque, and the souls of artistic photographers revolt from taking them. These accurate but unseemly portraits are, like the finger-prints, made in prisons.

Charts of Weight and Stature.—At the end of the book will be found nine Charts divided into squares for the periodical registration of Weight and Stature. Five of the charts are for the five five-yearly terms between birth and twenty-five years of age; the remaining four are summary charts, each for a twenty-five-yearly term. The five-yearly charts are divided into years and months by vertical lines one-twelfth of an inch apart; the twenty-five-yearly charts into years only, by lines one-fifth of an inch apart. The horizontal lines in both charts have the same meaning, and refer to the scales of inches and of pounds at their sides. Curves are printed in the charts intended for the period of development, which show the *average* weight and stature of the population of the British Isles. They are taken from the Report of a Committee (of which I was chairman) of the British Association in 1883. The figures are chiefly the result of the great industry of the late Mr. Charles Roberts. Sir R. Rawson also gave valuable assistance. The object of the curves is to enable the owner of the Album to detect any deviation from the normal in the sweep of his own curve. They are equally correct for all persons in their internal *proportions*, but by no means in their absolute values, as the different classes from whom the average is drawn differ widely among themselves. The average is too low for the professional and upper classes, too high for the very poor. It is also too low (other influences being the same) for the Scotch, too high for the Welsh, and so on. Thus the Report shows a difference in average stature in boys aged 11 to 12 years, in public schools and in industrial schools respectively, of almost exactly five inches (4.96), and that between the Scotch and Welsh generally, of three inches (2.97).

The importance of frequent observations of Weight and Stature in indicating latent mischief is greater than is commonly supposed. An arrested increase of weight, or, still more, the sudden loss of it, often precedes other symptoms of disease, and ought to draw attention to the health of the child. Insidious diseases may thus be discovered and withstood at their outset. The following diagram is drawn from one made by Professor H. P. Bowditch of Harvard University, U.S.A., and well illustrates the use of the weighing machine in warning approaching danger.

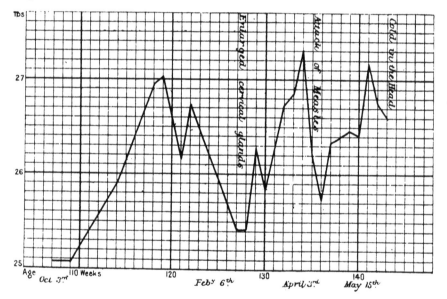

The observations were made every week upon a girl between the ages of two and three years. The first and prolonged loss of weight during December and January indicated a disorder of nutrition, which subsequently manifested itself by enlarged glands in the neck, and probably in the abdomen. Her health rapidly improved under treatment until March 27, when she again began to lose weight rapidly; this proved to be due to incipient measles, which appeared on April 5. She then gained weight up to May 15. Then a severe cold in the head caused her to lose weight again.

The scale of weights at the side of the charts ranges no higher than 160 lbs. (in other terms, than 11 stone 6 lbs.). When heavier weights than these have to be registered, a supplementary scale must be added, in which each of the side entries is increased by the even sum of 100 lbs.

Thus 160 will be written in the same line as 60, 200 on the same line as 100, and so on. There need be no confusion in consequence.

Parents of large and growing families would do well to purchase a weighing and measuring machine for the use of the household, occasionally testing its accuracy by putting known and heavy weights upon its platform.

The importance of variations of stature as a guide to health is also great, though not so great as that of weight. Times of unusually rapid growth are times when caution is needed. Physical and mental fatigue should be avoided during their occurrence, and for a while afterwards.

Records of Wife (or Husband).—A page is left at the end of the book on which the name and parentage of the wife (or husband) of the owner and the date of marriage may hereafter be written, together with other brief appropriate entries.

Records of Children.—Three pages are assigned to these; say, one page to the eldest child and half a page to each of four others in succession. More pages could be interleaved if wanted. A fresh Album ought to be started for each child.

Tests of Vision.—Simple forms of these, adequate for the present purpose, conclude the book.

See next page for

Genealogy of

RELATION.	BAPTISMAL NAME.	SURNAME.	PLACE OF BIRTH.	DATE.		
				DAY.	MONTH.	YEAR.
Self . . .						
Own Brothers .						
,, Sisters .						
Father . .						
Father's Father .						
,, Mother .						
Father's Brothers						
,, Sisters .						
Mother . .						
Mother's Father .						
,, Mother .						
Mother's Brothers						
,, Sisters .						

AGE AT DEATH.	CAUSE OF DEATH.	MINOR AILMENTS.

Characteristics common to two or more Members of the
Father's Family

Mother's Family

Description of Child at Birth

Name ....

Date of birth ....

Previous health of mother...

Birth at full time or premature ? ....

Labour natural or instrumental ? ....

* Physical peculiarities, if any (including " mother's marks ") ....

....

Weight at birth, after subtracting weight of clothes...

Length ....

Girth round nipples ....

† Colour of eyes, not at birth but a few days later...

Colour of hair, if any...

Child healthy or ailing ....

„   quiet or active...

„   feeble or vigorous ....

„   good tempered or fretful ....

* A verbatim copy of any record of strong mental impression, fright, shock, or fancy, occurring to the mother, which has been *written before the birth* of the child, should be added.

† The eyes of infants at birth are always dark blue.

Life and Medical History

1st YEAR

Life History

Medical History

2nd YEAR

Life History

Medical History

3rd YEAR

Life History

Medical History

Life and Medical History

Life History

Medical History

Life History

Medical History

Space for remarks, if any

Photographs taken between 0 and 5 Years of Age

Life and Medical History

END OF **6th** YEAR

Life History

Medical History

END OF **7th** YEAR

Life History

Medical History

END OF **8th** YEAR

Life History

Medical History

Life and Medical History

END OF **9th** YEAR

Life History

Medical History

END OF **10th** YEAR

Life History

Medical History

Space for Remarks, if any

Space for Remarks, if any

Anthropometric

	END OF **6th** YEAR.				END OF **7th** YEAR.			
Colour of eyes								
Colour of hair								
Other data								
	Test I.		Test II.		Test I.		Test II.	

	Test I.	Test II.	Test I.	Test II.
Sight — Right eye				
Sight — Left eye				
Sight — Colour vision				

	Self.	Three Others.			Self.	Three Others.		
		1	2	3		1	2	3
Hearing — Right ear	Self.	1	2	3	Self.	1	2	3
Hearing — Left ear	Self.	1	2	3	Self.	1	2	3

	Smell.	Taste.	Touch.	Smell.	Taste.	Touch.
Other senses						

	END OF 6th YEAR.	END OF 7th YEAR.
Teeth — Upper		
Teeth — Lower		
Mention any recent trial of bodily strength or endurance (long walk, etc.)		
Mention any recent trial of mental power (hard intellectual work)		
Mention any proof of marked artistic capacity		
Note any recently observed resemblances to others of the family, in features or in illnesses, at corresponding ages		
Additional Remarks		

Observations *(see* Letter-press for explanations)

END OF **8th** YEAR.		END OF **9th** YEAR.		END OF **10th** YEAR.	
Test I.	Test II.	Test I.	Test II.	Test I.	Test II.

Self.	Three Others.			Self.	Three Others.			Self.	Three Others.		
	I	2	3		I	2	3		I	2	3

Self.	Three Others.			Self.	Three Others.			Self.	Three Others.		
	I	2	3		I	2	3		I	2	3

Smell.	Taste.	Touch.	Smell.	Taste.	Touch.	Smell.	Taste.	Touch.

Photographs taken between 5 and 10 Years of Age

Life and Medical History

Life History

Medical History

END OF 12th YEAR

Life History

Medical History

END OF 13th YEAR

Life History

Medical History

Life and Medical History

END OF 14th YEAR

Life History

Medical History

END OF 15th YEAR

Life History

Medical History

Space for Remarks, if any

Space for Remarks, if any

Anthropometric

	END OF 11th YEAR.		END OF 12th YEAR.	
Colour of eyes				
Colour of hair				
Other data				
	Test I.	Test II.	Test I.	Test II.
Sight — Right eye				
Left eye				
Colour vision				
	Self.	Three Others. 1 2 3	Self.	Three Others. 1 2 3
Hearing — Right ear				
Left ear	Self.	Three Others. 1 2 3	Self.	Three Others. 1 2 3
Other senses	Smell. Taste. Touch.		Smell. Taste. Touch.	
Teeth — Upper				
Lower				
Mention any recent trial of bodily strength or endurance (long walk, etc.)				
Mention any recent trial of mental power (hard intellectual work)				
Mention any proof of marked artistic capacity				
Note any recently observed resemblances to others of the family, in features or in illnesses, at corresponding ages				
Additional remarks				

Observations *(see* Letter-press for explanations)

End of 13th Year.		End of 14th Year.		End of 15th Year.	

Test I.	Test II.	Test I.	Test II.	Test I.	Test II.

Self.	Three Others.			Self.	Three Others.			Self.	Three Others.		
	1	2	3		1	2	3		1	2	3

Self.	Three Others.			Self.	Three Others.			Self.	Three Others.		
	1	2	3		1	2	3		1	2	3

Smell.	Taste.	Touch.	Smell.	Taste.	Touch.	Smell.	Taste.	Touch.

Photographs taken between 10 and 15 Years of Age

Life and Medical History

END OF **16th** YEAR

Life History

Medical History

END OF **17th** YEAR

Life History

Medical History

END OF **18th** YEAR

Life History

Medical History

Life and Medical History

END OF **19th** YEAR

Life History

Medical History

END OF **20th** YEAR

Life History

Medical History

Space for Remarks, if any

Space for Remarks, if any

Anthropometric

	END OF **16th** YEAR.		END OF **17th** YEAR.	
Colour of eyes				
Colour of hair				
Other data				
	Test I.	Test II.	Test I.	Test II.
Sight — Right eye				
Sight — Left eye				
Sight — Colour vision . . .				

	Self.	Three Others.			Self.	Three Others.		
		1	2	3		1	2	3
Hearing — Right ear . . .								
Hearing — Left ear . . .								

	Smell.	Taste.	Touch.	Smell.	Taste.	Touch.
Other senses						

	END OF 16th YEAR.	END OF 17th YEAR.
Teeth — Upper		
Teeth — Lower		
Mention any recent trial of bodily strength or endurance (long walk, etc.)		
Mention any recent trial of mental power (hard intellectual work)		
Mention any proof of marked artistic capacity		
Note any recently observed resemblances to others of the family, in features or in illnesses, at corresponding ages		
Additional Remarks		

Observations (*see* Letter-press for explanations)

END OF **18th** YEAR.		END OF **19th** YEAR.		END OF **20th** YEAR.	
Test I.	Test II.	Test I.	Test II.	Test I.	Test II.

Self.	Three Others.			Self.	Three Others.			Self.	Three Others.		
	1	2	3		1	2	3		1	2	3

Self.	Three Others.			Self.	Three Others.			Self.	Three Others.		
	1	2	3		1	2	3		1	2	3

Smell.	Taste.	Touch.	Smell.	Taste.	Touch.	Smell.	Taste.	Touch.

Photographs taken between 15 and 20 Years of Age

Life and Medical History

END OF **21st** YEAR

Life History

Medical History

END OF **22nd** YEAR

Life History

Medical History

END OF **23rd** YEAR

Life History

Medical History

Life and Medical History

END OF **24th** YEAR

Life History

Medical History

END OF **25th** YEAR

Life History

Medical History

Space for Remarks, if any

Space for Remarks, if any

Anthropometric

	END OF **21st** YEAR.		END OF **22nd** YEAR.	
Colour of eyes				
Colour of hair				
Other data				
	Test I.	Test II.	Test I.	Test II.
Sight { Right eye . . .				
Left eye . . .				
Colour vision . .				
	Self. — Three Others. 1 2 3		Self. — Three Others. 1 2 3	
Hearing { Right ear . .				
Left ear . .	Self. — Three Others. 1 2 3		Self. — Three Others. 1 2 3	
	Smell. Taste. Touch.		Smell. Taste. Touch.	
Other senses				
Teeth { Upper . . .				
Lower . . .				
Mention any recent trial of bodily strength or endurance (long walk, etc.)				
Mention any recent trial of mental power (hard intellectual work)				
Mention any proof of marked artistic capacity				
Note any recently observed resemblances to others of the family, in features or in illnesses, at corresponding ages				
Additional remarks . . .				

Observations (*see* Letter-press for explanations)

END OF 23rd YEAR.				END OF 24th YEAR.				END OF 25th YEAR.			
Test I.		Test II.		Test I.		Test II.		Test I.		Test II.	
Self.	Three Others.			Self.	Three Others.			Self.	Three Others.		
	1	2	3		1	2	3		1	2	3
Self.	Three Others.			Self.	Three Others.			Self.	Three Others.		
	1	2	3		1	2	3		1	2	3
Smell.	Taste.	Touch.		Smell.	Taste.	Touch.		Smell.	Taste.	Touch.	

Photographs taken between **20** and **25** Years of Age

Life and Medical History

 END OF **26th** YEAR

Life History

Medical History

 END OF **27th** YEAR

Life History

Medical History

END OF **28th** YEAR

Life History

Medical History

Life and Medical History

 END OF **29th** YEAR

Life History

Medical History

 END OF **30th** YEAR

Life History

Medical History

Space for Remarks, if any

Space for Remarks, if any

Anthropometric

	END OF **26th** YEAR.		END OF **27th** YEAR.	
Colour of eyes				
Colour of hair				
Other data				
	Test I.	Test II.	Test I.	Test II.
Sight — Right eye . . .				
Left eye . . .				
Colour vision . . .				

Hearing — Right ear . . .	Self.	Three Others. 1 2 3	Self.	Three Others. 1 2 3
Left ear . . .	Self.	Three Others. 1 2 3	Self.	Three Others. 1 2 3

Other senses	Smell.	Taste.	Touch.	Smell.	Taste.	Touch.

Teeth — Upper		
Lower		

Mention any recent trial of bodily strength or endurance (long walk, etc.)		
Mention any recent trial of mental power (hard intellectual work)		
Mention any proof of marked artistic capacity		
Note any recently observed resemblances to others of the family, in features or in illnesses, at corresponding ages		
Additional Remarks		

Observations *(see* Letter-press for explanations)

End of **28th** Year.			End of **29th** Year.			End of **30th** Year.		
Test I.		Test II.	Test I.		Test II.	Test I.		Test II.

Self.	Three Others.			Self.	Three Others.			Self.	Three Others.		
	1	2	3		1	2	3		1	2	3

Self.	Three Others.			Self.	Three Others.			Self.	Three Others.		
	1	2	3		1	2	3		1	2	3

Smell.	Taste.	Touch.	Smell.	Taste.	Touch.	Smell.	Taste.	Touch.

Photographs taken between **25** and **30** Years of Age

Life and Medical History

Life History

Medical History

Life History

Medical History

Life History

Medical History

Life and Medical History

END OF **34th** YEAR

Life History

Medical History

END OF **35th** YEAR

Life History

Medical History

Space for Remarks, if any

Space for Remarks, if any

Anthropometric

	END OF **31st** YEAR.		END OF **32nd** YEAR.	
Colour of eyes				
Colour of hair				
Other data				

		Test I.	Test II.	Test I.	Test II.
Sight	Right eye				
	Left eye				
	Colour vision . .				

		Self.	Three Others.			Self.	Three Others.		
			1	2	3		1	2	3
Hearing	Right ear . . .								
	Left ear . . .	Self.	1	2	3	Self.	1	2	3

	Smell.	Taste.	Touch.	Smell.	Taste.	Touch.
Other senses						

Teeth	Upper			
	Lower			

Mention any recent trial of bodily strength or endurance (long walk, etc.)

Mention any recent trial of mental power (hard intellectual work)

Mention any proof of marked artistic capacity

Note any recently observed resemblances to others of the family, in features or in illnesses, at corresponding ages

Additional remarks . . . .

Observations *(see* Letter-press for explanations)

END OF **33rd** YEAR.			END OF **34th** YEAR.			END OF **35th** YEAR.		

Test I.	Test II.	Test I.	Test II.	Test I.	Test II.

Self.	Three Others.			Self.	Three Others.			Self.	Three Others.		
	1	2	3		1	2	3		1	2	3

Self.	Three Others.			Self.	Three Others.			Self.	Three Others.		
	1	2	3		1	2	3		1	2	3

Smell.	Taste.	Touch.	Smell.	Taste.	Touch.	Smell.	Taste.	Touch.

Photographs taken between 30 and 35 Years of Age

Life and Medical History

END OF **36th** YEAR

Life History

Medical History

END OF **37th** YEAR

Life History

Medical History

END OF **38th** YEAR

Life History

Medical History

Life and Medical History

Life History

Medical History

Life History

Medical History

Space for Remarks, if any

Space for Remarks, if any

Anthropometric

	END OF **36th** YEAR.		END OF **37th** YEAR.	
Colour of eyes				
Colour of hair				
Other data				
	Test I.	Test II.	Test I.	Test II.
Sight — Right eye				
Sight — Left eye				
Sight — Colour vision . . .				

		END OF 36th YEAR				END OF 37th YEAR		
	Self.	Three Others.			Self.	Three Others.		
Hearing — Right ear . .		1	2	3		1	2	3
	Self.	Three Others.			Self.	Three Others.		
Hearing — Left ear . .		1	2	3		1	2	3

	Smell.	Taste.	Touch.	Smell.	Taste.	Touch.
Other senses						

	END OF 36th YEAR	END OF 37th YEAR
Teeth — Upper		
Teeth — Lower		
Mention any recent trial of bodily strength or endurance (long walk, etc.)		
Mention any recent trial of mental power (hard intellectual work)		
Mention any proof of marked artistic capacity		
Note any recently observed resemblances to others of the family, in features or in illnesses, at corresponding ages		
Additional Remarks		

Observations (*see* Letter-press for explanations)

END OF **38th** YEAR.			END OF **39th** YEAR.			END OF **40th** YEAR.		

Test I.	Test II.		Test I.	Test II.		Test I.	Test II.	

Self.	Three Others.			Self.	Three Others.			Self.	Three Others.		
	1	2	3		1	2	3		1	2	3

Self.	Three Others.			Self.	Three Others.			Self.	Three Others.		
	1	2	3		1	2	3		1	2	3

Smell.	Taste.	Touch.	Smell.	Taste.	Touch.	Smell.	Taste.	Touch.

Photographs taken between 35 and 40 Years of Age

Life and Medical History

Life History

Medical History

Life History

Medical History

Life History

Medical History

Life and Medical History

END OF **44th** YEAR

Life History

Medical History

END OF **45th** YEAR

Life History

Medical History

Space for Remarks, if any

Space for Remarks, if any

Anthropometric

	END OF 41st YEAR.		END OF 42nd YEAR.	
Colour of eyes				
Colour of hair				
Other data				

	Test I.	Test II.	Test I.	Test II.
Sight { Right eye				
Left eye				
Colour vision . . .				

	Self.	Three Others.			Self.	Three Others.		
		1	2	3		1	2	3
Hearing { Right ear . . .								
	Self.	Three Others.			Self.	Three Others.		
		1	2	3		1	2	3
Left ear . . .								

	Smell.	Taste.	Touch.	Smell.	Taste.	Touch.
Other senses						

Teeth { Upper		
Lower		
Mention any recent trial of bodily strength or endurance (long walk, etc.)		
Mention any recent trial of mental power (hard intellectual work)		
Mention any proof of marked artistic capacity		
Note any recently observed resemblances to others of the family, in features or in illnesses, at corresponding ages		
Additional remarks		

Observations (*see* Letter-press for explanations)

END OF **43rd** YEAR.		END OF **44th** YEAR.		END OF **45th** YEAR.	

Test I.	Test II.	Test I.	Test II.	Test I.	Test II.

Self.	Three Others.			Self.	Three Others.			Self.	Three Others.		
	1	2	3		1	2	3		1	2	3

Self.	Three Others.			Self.	Three Others.			Self.	Three Others.		
	1	2	3		1	2	3		1	2	3

Smell.	Taste.	Touch.	Smell.	Taste.	Touch.	Smell.	Taste.	Touch.

Photographs taken between **40** and **45** Years of Age

Life and Medical History

END OF **46th** YEAR

Life History

Medical History

END OF **47th** YEAR

Life History

Medical History

END OF **48th** YEAR

Life History

Medical History

H

Life and Medical History

END OF **49th** YEAR

Life History

Medical History

END OF **50th** YEAR

Life History

Medical History

Space for Remarks, if any

Space for Remarks, if any

Anthropometric

	END OF **46th** YEAR.				END OF **47th** YEAR.			
Colour of eyes								
Colour of hair								
Other data								

		Test I.	Test II.		Test I.	Test II.		
Sight	Right eye							
	Left eye							
	Colour vision . . .							

		Self.	Three Others.			Self.	Three Others.		
			1	2	3		1	2	3
Hearing	Right ear . .								
	Left ear . . .	Self.	1	2	3	Self.	1	2	3

	Smell.	Taste.	Touch.	Smell.	Taste.	Touch.
Other senses						

Teeth	Upper		
	Lower		

	END OF 46th YEAR	END OF 47th YEAR
Mention any recent trial of bodily strength or endurance (long walk, etc.)		
Mention any recent trial of mental power (hard intellectual work)		
Mention any proof of marked artistic capacity		
Note any recently observed resemblances to others of the family, in features or in illnesses, at corresponding ages		
Additional Remarks		

Observations (*see* Letter-press for explanations)

END OF 48th YEAR.		END OF 49th YEAR.		END OF 50th YEAR.	
Test I.	Test II.	Test I.	Test II.	Test I.	Test II.

Self.	Three Others.			Self.	Three Others.			Self.	Three Others.		
	1	2	3		1	2	3		1	2	3

Self.	Three Others.			Self.	Three Others.			Self.	Three Others.		
	1	2	3		1	2	3		1	2	3

Smell.	Taste.	Touch.	Smell.	Taste.	Touch.	Smell.	Taste.	Touch.

Photographs taken between 45 and 50 Years of Age

Life and Medical History

END OF **51st** YEAR

Life History

Medical History

END OF **52nd** YEAR

Life History

Medical History

END OF **53rd** YEAR

Life History

Medical History

Life and Medical History

END OF **54th** YEAR

Life History

Medical History

END OF **55th** YEAR

Life History

Medical History

Space for Remarks, if any

Space for Remarks, if any

Anthropometric

	END OF **51st** YEAR.		END OF **52nd** YEAR.	
Colour of eyes				
Colour of hair				
Other data				
	Test I.	Test II.	Test I.	Test II.
Sight — Right eye				
Left eye				
Colour vision . . .				

	Self.	Three Others. 1 2 3	Self.	Three Others. 1 2 3
Hearing — Right ear . . .				
Left ear . . .	Self.	Three Others. 1 2 3	Self.	Three Others. 1 2 3

	Smell.	Taste.	Touch.	Smell.	Taste.	Touch.
Other senses						

Teeth — Upper . . .		
Lower . . .		
Mention any recent trial of bodily strength or endurance (long walk, etc.)		
Mention any recent trial of mental power (hard intellectual work)		
Mention any proof of marked artistic capacity		
Note any recently observed resemblances to others of the family, in features or in illnesses, at corresponding ages		
Additional remarks		

Observations (*see* Letter-press for explanations)

END OF **53rd** YEAR.		END OF **54th** YEAR.		END OF **55th** YEAR.	

Test I.	Test II.	Test I.	Test II.	Test I.	Test II.

Self.	Three Others.			Self.	Three Others.			Self.	Three Others.		
	I	2	3		I	2	3		I	2	3

Self.	Three Others.			Self.	Three Others.			Self.	Three Others.		
	I	2	3		I	2	3		I	2	3

Smell.	Taste.	Touch.	Smell.	Taste.	Touch.	Smell.	Taste.	Touch.

Photographs taken between 50 and 55 Years of Age

Life and Medical History

END OF **56th** YEAR

Life History

Medical History

END OF **57th** YEAR

Life History

Medical History

END OF **58th** YEAR

Life History

Medical History

Life and Medical History

END OF **59th** YEAR

Life History

Medical History

END OF **60th** YEAR

Life History

Medical History

Space for Remarks, if any

Space for Remarks, if any

Anthropometric

	END OF 56th YEAR.				END OF 57th YEAR.			
Colour of eyes								
Colour of hair								
Other data								

	Test I.	Test II.		Test I.	Test II.	
Sight { Right eye . . .						
Left eye . . .						
Colour vision . .						

	Self.	Three Others.			Self.	Three Others.		
		1	2	3		1	2	3
Hearing { Right ear . .								
Left ear . . .	Self.	1	2	3	Self.	1	2	3

	Smell.	Taste.	Touch.	Smell.	Taste.	Touch.
Other senses						

Teeth { Upper		
Lower		
Mention any recent trial of bodily strength or endurance (long walk, etc.)		
Mention any recent trial of mental power (hard intellectual work)		
Mention any proof of marked artistic capacity		
Note any recently observed resemblances to others of the family, in features or in illnesses, at corresponding ages		
Additional Remarks		

Observations (*see* Letter-press for explanations)

END OF **58th** YEAR.		END OF **59th** YEAR.		END OF **60th** YEAR.	
Test I.	Test II.	Test I.	Test II.	Test I.	Test II.

Self.	Three Others.			Self.	Three Others.			Self.	Three Others.		
	1	2	3		1	2	3		1	2	3

Self.	Three Others.			Self.	Three Others.			Self.	Three Others.		
	1	2	3		1	2	3		1	2	3

Smell.	Taste.	Touch.	Smell.	Taste.	Touch.	Smell.	Taste.	Touch.

Photographs taken between 55 and 60 Years of Age

Life and Medical History

END OF **61st** YEAR

Life History

Medical History

END OF **62nd** YEAR

Life History

Medical History

END OF **63rd** YEAR

Life History

Medical History

Life and Medical History

END OF **64th** YEAR

Life History

Medical History

END OF **65th** YEAR

Life History

Medical History

Space for Remarks, if any

Space for Remarks, if any

Anthropometric

	END OF **61st** YEAR.		END OF **62nd** YEAR.	
Colour of eyes				
Colour of hair				
Other data				
	Test I.	Test II.	Test I.	Test II.
Sight { Right eye . . .				
Left eye . . .				
Colour vision . . .				
	Self.	Three Others. 1 2 3	Self.	Three Others. 1 2 3
Hearing { Right ear . .				
Left ear . .	Self.	Three Others. 1 2 3	Self.	Three Others. 1 2 3
	Smell.	Taste.	Touch.	Smell.	Taste.	Touch.
Other senses				
Teeth { Upper . . .				
Lower . . .				
Mention any recent trial of bodily strength or endurance (long walk, etc.)				
Mention any recent trial of mental power (hard intellectual work)				
Mention any proof of marked artistic capacity				
Note any recently observed resemblances to others of the family, in features or in illnesses, at corresponding ages				
Additional remarks . . .				

Observations (*see* Letter-press for explanations)

END OF **63rd** YEAR.	END OF **64th** YEAR.	END OF **65th** YEAR.

Test I.	Test II.	Test I.	Test II.	Test I.	Test II.

Self.	Three Others.			Self.	Three Others.			Self.	Three Others.		
	1	2	3		1	2	3		1	2	3

Self.	Three Others.			Self.	Three Others.			Self.	Three Others.		
	1	2	3		1	2	3		1	2	3

Smell.	Taste.	Touch.	Smell.	Taste.	Touch.	Smell.	Taste.	Touch.

Photographs taken between 60 and 65 Years of Age

Life and Medical History

END OF **66th** YEAR

Life History

Medical History

END OF **67th** YEAR

Life History

Medical History

END OF **68th** YEAR

Life History

Medical History

Life and Medical History

END OF **69th** YEAR

Life History

Medical History

END OF **70th** YEAR

Life History

Medical History

Space for Remarks, if any

Space for Remarks, if any

Anthropometric

	END OF 66th YEAR.			END OF 67th YEAR.		
Colour of eyes						
Colour of hair						
Other data						

	Test I.	Test II.		Test I.	Test II.	
Sight — Right eye						
Left eye						
Colour vision						

	Self.	Three Others. 1 2 3		Self.	Three Others. 1 2 3	
Hearing — Right ear						
Left ear						

	Smell.	Taste.	Touch.	Smell.	Taste.	Touch.
Other senses						

Teeth — Upper						
Lower						
Mention any recent trial of bodily strength or endurance (long walk, etc.)						
Mention any recent trial of mental power (hard intellectual work)						
Mention any proof of marked artistic capacity						
Note any recently observed resemblances to others of the family, in features or in illnesses, at corresponding ages						
Additional Remarks						

Observations (*see* Letter-press for explanations)

END OF **68th** YEAR.		END OF **69th** YEAR.		END OF **70th** YEAR.	
Test I.	Test II.	Test I.	Test II.	Test I.	Test II.

Self.	Three Others.			Self.	Three Others.			Self.	Three Others.		
	1	2	3		1	2	3		1	2	3
Self.	Three Others.			Self.	Three Others.			Self.	Three Others.		
	1	2	3		1	2	3		1	2	3

Smell.	Taste.	Touch.	Smell.	Taste.	Touch.	Smell.	Taste.	Touch.

Photographs taken between 65 and 70 Years of Age

Life and Medical History

END OF **71st** YEAR

Life History

Medical History

END OF **72nd** YEAR

Life History

Medical History

END OF **73rd** YEAR

Life History

Medical History

Life and Medical History

Life History   END OF **74th** YEAR

Medical History

Life History   END OF **75th** YEAR

Medical History

Space for Remarks, if any

Space for Remarks, if any

Anthropometric

	END OF **71st** YEAR.		END OF **72nd** YEAR.	
Colour of eyes				
Colour of hair				
Other data				
	Test I.	Test II.	Test I.	Test II.
Sight — Right eye				
Left eye				
Colour vision . .				
	Self.	Three Others. 1 2 3	Self.	Three Others. 1 2 3
Hearing — Right ear . .				
Left ear . . .	Self.	Three Others. 1 2 3	Self.	Three Others. 1 2 3
Other senses	Smell. Taste. Touch.		Smell. Taste. Touch.	
Teeth — Upper				
Lower				
Mention any recent trial of bodily strength or endurance (long walk, etc.)				
Mention any recent trial of mental power (hard intellectual work)				
Mention any proof of marked artistic capacity				
Note any recently observed resemblances to others of the family, in features or in illnesses, at corresponding ages				
Additional remarks				

Observations (*see* Letter-press for explanations)

END OF **73rd** YEAR.				END OF **74th** YEAR.				END OF **75th** YEAR.			
Test I.		Test II.		Test I.		Test II.		Test I.		Test II.	

Self.	Three Others.			Self.	Three Others.			Self.	Three Others.		
	1	2	3		1	2	3		1	2	3

Self.	Three Others.			Self.	Three Others.			Self.	Three Others.		
	1	2	3		1	2	3		1	2	3

Smell.	Taste.	Touch.	Smell.	Taste.	Touch.	Smell.	Taste.	Touch.

Photographs taken between 70 and 75 Years of Age

Life and Medical History

END OF **76th** YEAR

Life History

Medical History

END OF **77th** YEAR

Life History

Medical History

END OF **78th** YEAR

Life History

Medical History

Life and Medical History

END OF **79th** YEAR

Life History

Medical History

END OF **80th** YEAR

Life History

Medical History

Space for Remarks, if any

Space for Remarks, if any

Anthropometric

	END OF 76th YEAR.		END OF 77th YEAR.	
Colour of eyes				
Colour of hair				
Other data				
	Test I.	Test II.	Test I.	Test II.
Sight { Right eye . . .				
Left eye . . .				
Colour vision . . .				

		Self.	Three Others. 1 2 3	Self.	Three Others. 1 2 3
Hearing {	Right ear . .				
	Left ear . .	Self.	Three Others. 1 2 3	Self.	Three Others. 1 2 3

	Smell.	Taste.	Touch.	Smell.	Taste.	Touch.
Other senses . . .						

Teeth { Upper . . .			
Lower . . .			
Mention any recent trial of bodily strength or endurance (long walk, etc.)			
Mention any recent trial of mental power (hard intellectual work)			
Mention any proof of marked artistic capacity			
Note any recently observed resemblances to others of the family, in features or in illnesses, at corresponding ages			
Additional Remarks . . .			

Observations (*see* Letter-press for explanations)

END OF **78th** YEAR.	END OF **79th** YEAR.	END OF **80th** YEAR.

Test I.	Test II.	Test I.	Test II.	Test I.	Test II.

Self.	Three Others.			Self.	Three Others.			Self.	Three Others.		
	I	2	3		I	2	3		I	2	3

Self.	Three Others.			Self.	Three Others.			Self.	Three Others.		
	I	2	3		I	2	3		I	2	3

Smell.	Taste.	Touch.	Smell.	Taste.	Touch.	Smell.	Taste.	Touch.

Photographs taken between 75 and 80 Years of Age

Life and Medical History

END OF **81st** YEAR

Life History

Medical History

END OF **82nd** YEAR

Life History

Medical History

END OF **83rd** YEAR

Life History

Medical History

Life and Medical History

END OF **84th** YEAR

Life History

Medical History

END OF **85th** YEAR

Life History

Medical History

Space for Remarks, if any

Space for Remarks, if any

Anthropometric

			END OF **81st** YEAR.				END OF **82nd** YEAR.			
Colour of eyes										
Colour of hair										
Other data										
			Test I.		Test II.		Test I.		Test II.	
Sight	Right eye . . .									
	Left eye . . .									
	Colour vision . .									
			Self.	Three Others.			Self.	Three Others.		
				1	2	3		1	2	3
Hearing	Right ear . .									
	Left ear . .	Self.	Three Others.			Self.	Three Others.			
			1	2	3		1	2	3	
Other senses		Smell.	Taste.		Touch.	Smell.	Taste.		Touch.	
Teeth	Upper . . .									
	Lower . . .									
Mention any recent trial of bodily strength or endurance (long walk, etc.)										
Mention any recent trial of mental power (hard intellectual work)										
Mention any proof of marked artistic capacity										
Note any recently observed resemblances to others of the family, in features or in illnesses, at corresponding ages										
Additional remarks . . .										

Observations (*see* Letter-press for explanations)

END OF 83rd YEAR.		END OF 84th YEAR.		END OF 85th YEAR.	
Test I.	Test II.	Test I.	Test II.	Test I.	Test II.
Self.	Three Others.	Self.	Three Others.	Self.	Three Others.
	1　　2　　3		1　　2　　3		1　　2　　3
Self.	Three Others.	Self.	Three Others.	Self.	Three Others.
	1　　2　　3		1　　2　　3		1　　2　　3
Smell.	Taste.	Touch.	Smell.	Taste.	Touch.

Photographs taken between 80 and 85 Years of Age

Life and Medical History

END OF **86th** YEAR

Life History

Medical History

END OF **87th** YEAR

Life History

Medical History

END OF **88th** YEAR

Life History

Medical History

Life and Medical History

END OF **89th** YEAR

Life History

Medical History

END OF **90th** YEAR

Life History

Medical History

Space for Remarks, if any

Space for Remarks, if any

Anthropometric

	END OF **86th** YEAR.		END OF **87th** YEAR.	
Colour of eyes				
Colour of hair				
Other data				
	Test I.	Test II.	Test I.	Test II.
Sight — Right eye . . .				
Sight — Left eye . . .				
Sight — Colour vision . . .				
Hearing — Right ear . .	Self. — Three Others. 1 2 3		Self. — Three Others. 1 2 3	
Hearing — Left ear . . .	Self. — Three Others. 1 2 3		Self. — Three Others. 1 2 3	
Other senses	Smell. Taste. Touch.		Smell. Taste. Touch.	
Teeth — Upper				
Teeth — Lower				
Mention any recent trial of bodily strength or endurance (long walk, etc.)				
Mention any recent trial of mental power (hard intellectual work)				
Mention any proof of marked artistic capacity				
Note any recently observed resemblances to others of the family, in features or in illnesses, at corresponding ages				
Additional Remarks . . .				

Observations (*see* Letter-press for explanations)

END OF **88th** YEAR.		END OF **89th** YEAR.		END OF **90th** YEAR.	
Test I.	Test II.	Test I.	Test II.	Test I.	Test II.

Self.	Three Others.			Self.	Three Others.			Self.	Three Others.		
	I	2	3		I	2	3		I	2	3

Self.	Three Others.			Self.	Three Others.			Self.	Three Others.		
	I	2	3		I	2	3		I	2	3

Smell.	Taste.	Touch.	Smell.	Taste.	Touch.	Smell.	Taste.	Touch.

Photographs taken between 85 and 90 Years of Age

Life and Medical History

END OF **91st** YEAR

Life History

Medical History

END OF **92nd** YEAR

Life History

Medical History

END OF **93rd** YEAR

Life History

Medical History

Life and Medical History

END OF **94th** YEAR

Life History

Medical History

END OF **95th** YEAR

Life History

Medical History

Space for Remarks, if any

Space for Remarks, if any

Anthropometric

		END OF 91st YEAR.		END OF 92nd YEAR.	
Colour of eyes					
Colour of hair					
Other data					

		Test I.	Test II.	Test I.	Test II.
Sight	Right eye . . .				
	Left eye . . .				
	Colour vision . .				

		Self.	Three Others. 1 2 3	Self.	Three Others. 1 2 3
Hearing	Right ear . .				
	Left ear . .	Self.	Three Others. 1 2 3	Self.	Three Others. 1 2 3

		Smell.	Taste.	Touch.	Smell.	Taste.	Touch.
Other senses							

Teeth	Upper . . .		
	Lower . . .		

Mention any recent trial of bodily strength or endurance (long walk, etc.)		
Mention any recent trial of mental power (hard intellectual work)		
Mention any proof of marked artistic capacity		
Note any recently observed resemblances to others of the family, in features or in illnesses, at corresponding ages		
Additional remarks		

Observations *(see* Letter-press for explanations)

END OF **93rd** YEAR.			END OF **94th** YEAR.			END OF **95th** YEAR.		
Test I.	Test II.		Test I.	Test II.		Test I.	Test II.	
Self.	Three Others.		Self.	Three Others.		Self.	Three Others.	
	1	2	3		1	2	3		1	2	3
Self.	Three Others.		Self.	Three Others.		Self.	Three Others.	
	1	2	3		1	2	3		1	2	3
Smell.	Taste.	Touch.	Smell.	Taste.	Touch.	Smell.	Taste.	Touch.

Photographs taken between 90 and 95 Years of Age

Life and Medical History

END OF **96th** YEAR

Life History

Medical History

END OF **97th** YEAR

Life History

Medical History

END OF **98th** YEAR

Life History

Medical History

N

Life and Medical History

END OF **99th** YEAR

Life History

Medical History

END OF **100th** YEAR

Life History

Medical History

Space for Remarks, if any

Space for Remarks, if any

Anthropometric

	END OF **96th** YEAR.		END OF **97th** YEAR.	
Colour of eyes				
Colour of hair				
Other data				
	Test I.	Test II.	Test I.	Test II.
Sight { Right eye				
Left eye				
Colour vision . . .				

		Self.	Three Others.			Self.	Three Others.		
			1	2	3		1	2	3
Hearing { Right ear . . .									
Left ear . . .									

	Smell.	Taste.	Touch.	Smell.	Taste.	Touch.
Other senses						

Teeth { Upper		
Lower		
Mention any recent trial of bodily strength or endurance (long walk, etc.)		
Mention any recent trial of mental power (hard intellectual work)		
Mention any proof of marked artistic capacity		
Note any recently observed resemblances to others of the family, in features or in illnesses, at corresponding ages		
Additional Remarks		

Observations *(see* Letter-press for explanations)

END OF **98th** YEAR.		END OF **99th** YEAR.		END OF **100th** YEAR.	
Test I.	Test II.	Test I.	Test II.	Test I.	Test II.

Self.	Three Others.			Self.	Three Others.			Self.	Three Others.		
	1	2	3		1	2	3		1	2	3

Self.	Three Others.			Self.	Three Others.			Self.	Three Others.		
	1	2	3		1	2	3		1	2	3

Smell.	Taste.	Touch.	Smell.	Taste.	Touch.	Smell.	Taste.	Touch.

Photographs taken between 95 and 100 Years of Age

Records of Wife (or Husband)

Records of Children

Records of Children

Records of Children

APPENDIX

TESTS OF VISION

TEST TYPES FOR ACUTENESS OF VISION. (Test I.) *Distant Vision.*— Place this open page against a wall, at a distance of at least 15 feet, in good daylight. If you can read the annexed Test Type, No. 1, at this or at a greater distance, your vision is good. If you are unable to read it at 15 feet, then very gradually draw nearer, until you are able to do so, and note the distance in feet in the proper page and place.

LSEOFDTHUC

No. 1.

(Test II.) *Near Vision.*—The Test Type, No. 2, may be read by a person of average sight, in good daylight and without glasses, at a distance of 12 inches. If you are unable to do this, approach your eyes very gradually to the page until you are just able to read it accurately. Note the distance in inches in the appropriate page and place.

The Palace of Holyrood House stands at the eastern extremity of the city, and at the bottom of the Canongate. It is a beautiful building, of a quadrangular form, with an open court, which is ninety-four feet square. The more ancient parts of this fine edifice, consisting of the north-west towers, were re-built by James V. about the year 1528, though Holyrood seems to have been an occasional royal residence for ages before. During the minority of Queen Mary, the Palace of Holyrood was burnt, as well as the city, by the English forces under the Earl of Hertford; soon after, it was repaired and enlarged beyond its present size.

No. 2.

In case you are not able to read it at all, make a note to that effect.

TESTS FOR COLOUR VISION.—Procure a small heap of bits of variously coloured wools, and apply to some friend, who has the credit of being able to match colours well, to test you. As women are very rarely colour blind, the verdict of two ladies might be relied on. They should be asked to select a sample of distinctly green wool, and to request you to sort out of the rest of the heap, and to lay by the side of the sample, every bit of wool that has any tinge of green in it. The majority of the wools used for the test should be of delicate tints, and varieties of browns, pinks, reds, violets, yellows, greys, and greens. The trial should be made in good daylight, and it should be insisted upon that no clue nor guidance should be given to help you in your choice.

Printed by R. & R. CLARK, LIMITED, *Edinburgh.*

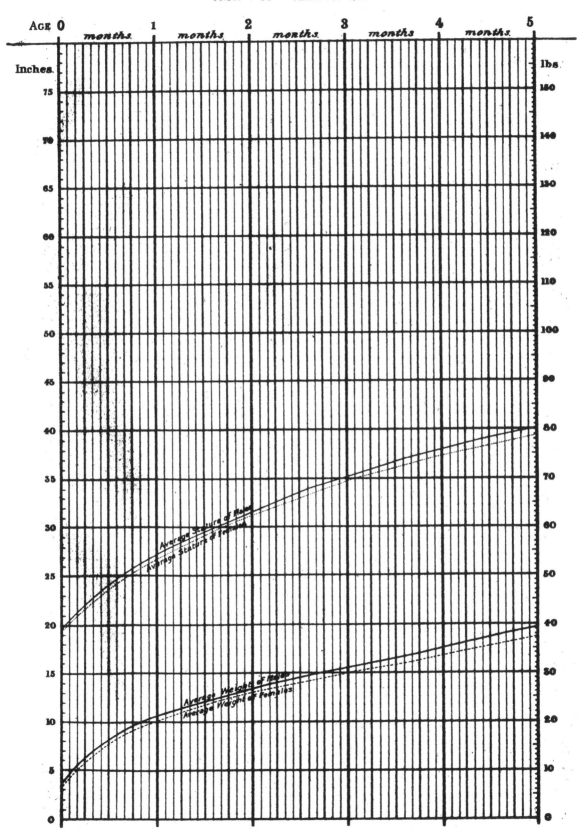

CHART I. ON WHICH TO RECORD WEIGHT AND STATURE FROM 0 TO 5 YEARS OF AGE.

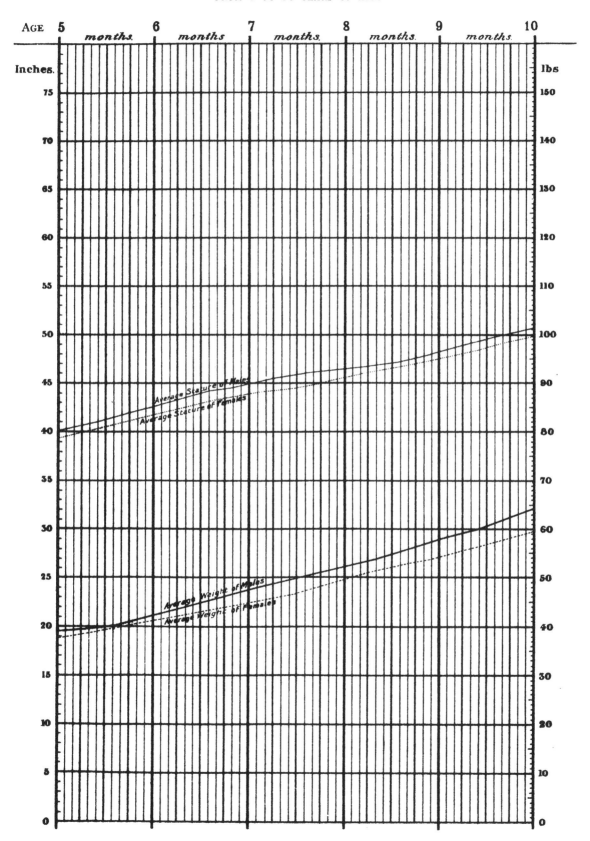

CHART II. ON WHICH TO RECORD WEIGHT AND STATURE
FROM 5 TO 10 YEARS OF AGE.

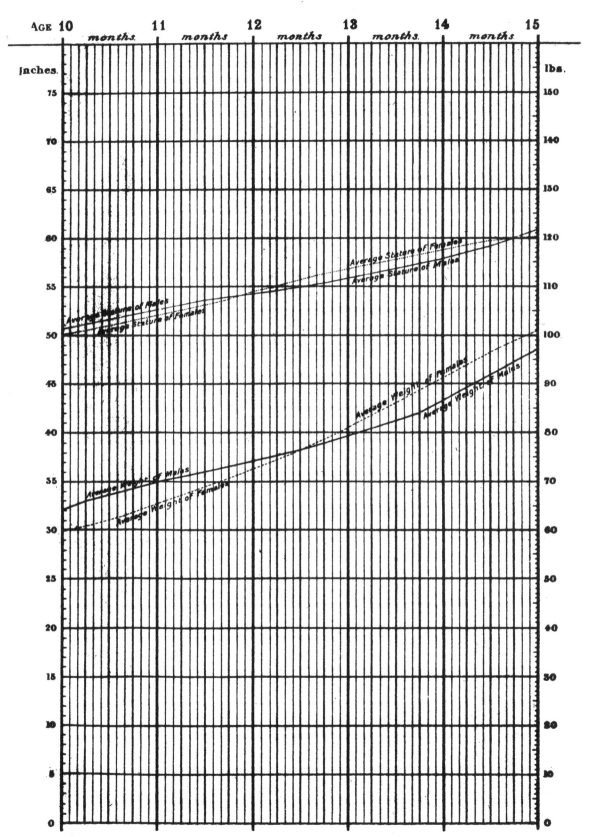

CHART III. ON WHICH TO RECORD WEIGHT AND STATURE
FROM 10 TO 15 YEARS OF AGE.

CHART IV. ON WHICH TO RECORD WEIGHT AND STATURE
FROM 15 TO 20 YEARS OF AGE.

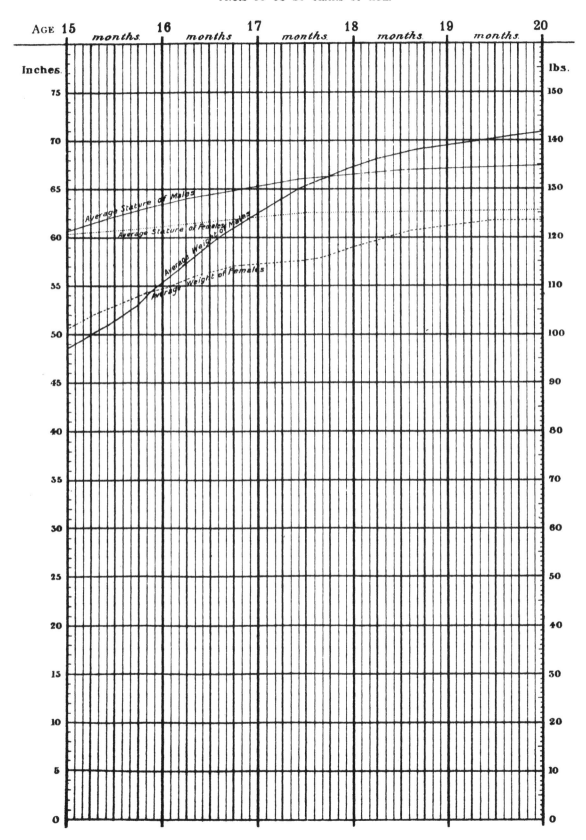

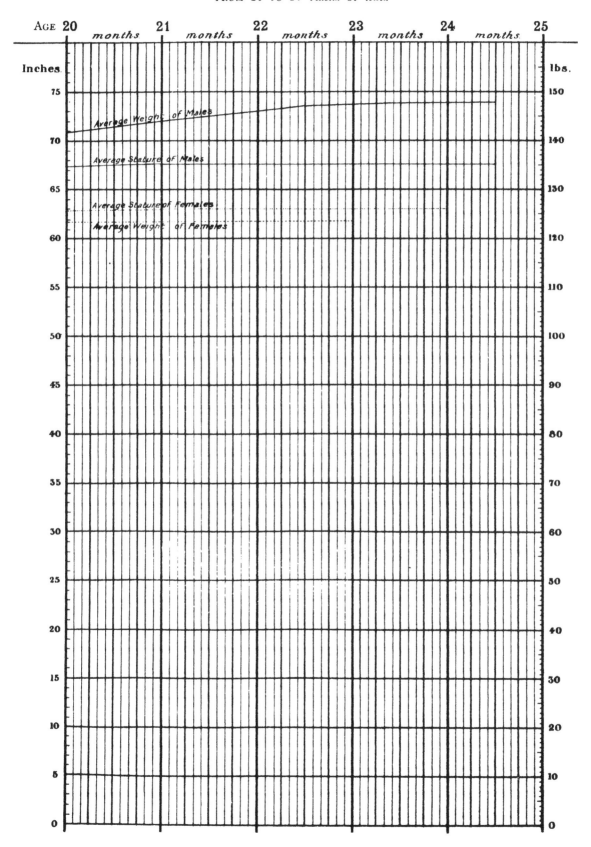

CHART V. ON WHICH TO RECORD WEIGHT AND STATURE
FROM 20 TO 25 YEARS OF AGE.

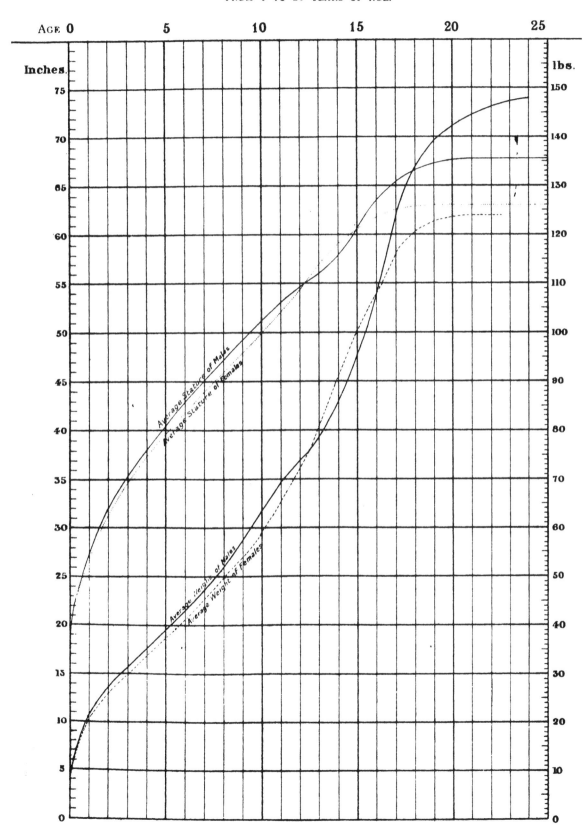

CHART VI. ON WHICH TO RECORD WEIGHT AND STATURE
FROM 0 TO 25 YEARS OF AGE.

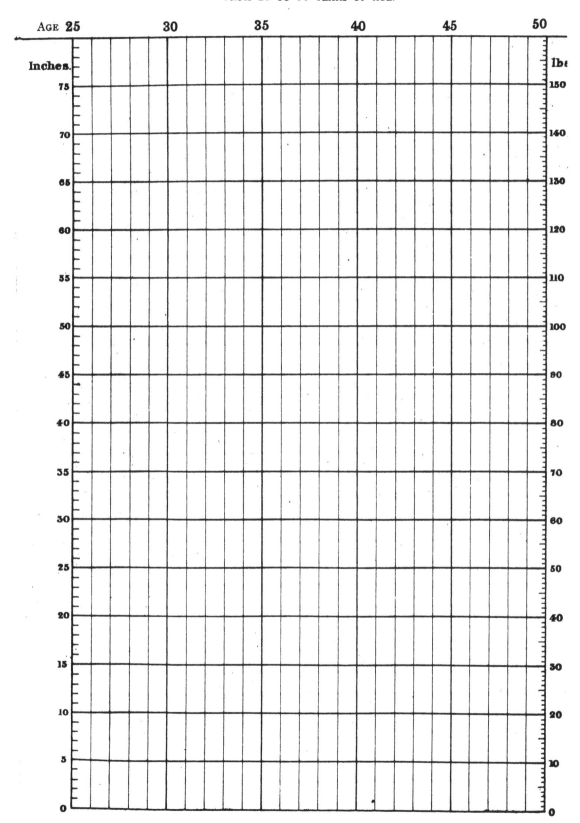

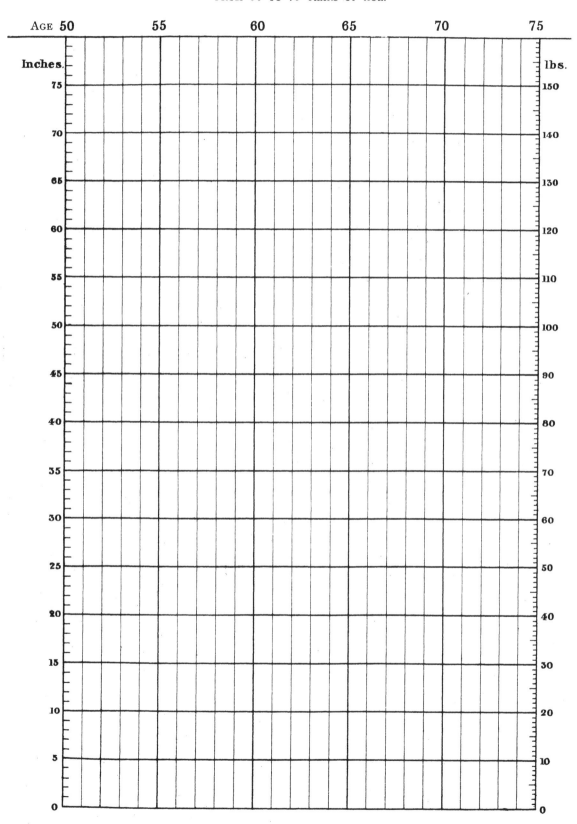

CHART VIII. ON WHICH TO RECORD WEIGHT AND STATURE
FROM 50 TO 75 YEARS OF AGE.

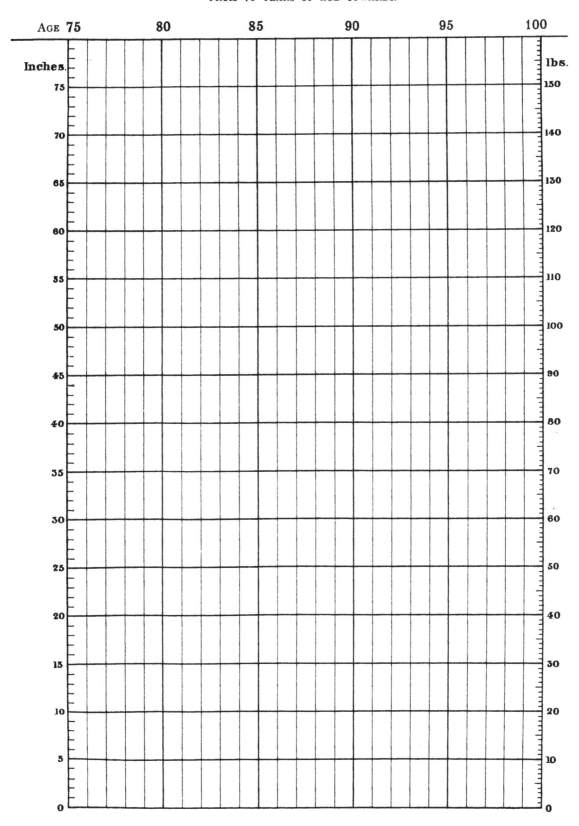

CHART IX. ON WHICH TO RECORD WEIGHT AND STATURE
FROM 75 YEARS OF AGE UPWARDS.